High Protein Diet

High Protein Everyday Meals for Metabolism Boost and Weight Loss

All Rights Reserved. No part of this publication may be reproduced in any form or by any means, including scanning, photocopying, or otherwise without prior written permission of the copyright holder. Copyright © 2014

Table of Contents

Introduction

Why Eat High Protein?

Foods to Avoid

High Protein Baking

Almond Butter Crunch Granola Bar
Vanilla Bean Shortbread Cookies
Cranberry Pistachio Biscotti
Super-Protein Coconut Custard Pie
Vanilla Peach Cake
Walnut Raisin Cookies
Indian Sweet Almond Fudge
Asian Sesame Cookies
Blueberry Scones
Classic Bagels
Avocado Club Muffin
Carrot Cake Cookie Bars

Ginger Spice Cookies
Rosemary Basil Scones
Cinnamon Cashew Rugalach
Kefir Sourdough Rolls
Chocolate Pecan Shortbread Cookies
Cocoa Gingerbread
State Fair Fry Bread
Easy Biscuits
Cranberry Pistachio Scones
Avocado Spice Bread
Apple Upside Down Cakes
Cashew Belgian Waffles
Fruit And Nut Cake
Chocolate Almond Biscotti
Wild Mince Meat Pie
High-Protein Pretzel Sticks
Slow Cooker Berry Cobbler
Avocado Club Muffin

High Protein Dinners

High Protein Chicken Satay
Saucy Meatballs
Crunchy Cashew Chicken
Thai Steamed Mussels
Steak and Eggs
Primal Chicken and Waffles
Southern Style Egg Salad
Meaty Texas Chili
Almond Crust Chicken Pie
Nuts & Turkey Burgers
Baked Tilapia Filets
Super Simple Protein Matzo Ball Soup
Highland Beef Haggis
Bacon Wrapped Filet Mignon
Herb Crusted Pork Chops with Cinnamon Apples
Sausage Stuffed Tomatoes
Stuffed Cabbage in Tomato Sauce
Beef Burgundy
Delicious Lobster Bisque

Stewed Chicken and Dumplings
Macadamia Crusted Ahi Tuna
Lobster Newburg
Island Lamb Patty
Jamaican Curried Goat
Holiday Baked Ham
Chickplant Filets
Salmon with Berry Chutney
Oven-Fried Chicken
Country Fried Steak
Southern Liver and Onions

Why Eat High Protein?

Contrary to popular belief, a high-protein diet doesn't necessarily equal a low-carb or ketogenic diet. Protein acts like "building blocks" which your body disassembles and reassembles as needed. A protein is nothing more than a long chain of amino acids. Protein is said to be "complete" when it contains all 9 of the essential amino acids, and "incomplete" when it lacks one or more essential amino acid. These amino acids are essential because our body cannot produce them and they have to be consumed through food. Animal-sourced protein is usually complete while plant-based protein is often incomplete. This does not make plant-based protein inferior – it only means you need to vary your protein sources in order to receive a healthy dose of all the essential amino acids.

High protein diets are popular among very active people, who need astonishing amounts of protein to support their physical activity. For example, bodybuilders often need to eat high amounts of protein just to build and regenerate muscle. For the regular person, a high protein diet may help lose fat by reducing consumption of carbs, which are often linked to weight gain. Because protein contains the same amount of calories per gram when compared to carbs, it is wise to limit protein intake to reasonable amounts. This means replacing carbs with protein and not just adding more protein to your diet. For this reason, when fitting a high-protein diet in a calorie budget, it is preferable to eliminate carbs and starchy foods in favour of protein. Going over your daily calorie goal could still lead to weight gain, even if the foods are protein-based.

Protein is essential for energy levels, tissue and muscle repair and general health maintenance. Not eating enough protein can lead to fatigue and muscle loss. This is especially important for vegetarians and vegans, who can become protein-deficient quickly if not careful due to not eating meat or other animal protein. Fitting high-protein foods in your regular diet will help you feel fuller longer and give you an edge when it comes to resisting food cravings. Carbs cause blood sugar to rise and fall quickly, while protein tends to keep blood sugar more stable as it is digested slowly. This means that a high-protein diet can help you lose weight and reduce the effect of insulin resistance. Just make sure to always include some healthy fats, as well as some healthy carbs (fruits and veggies) if not trying to get into ketosis.

Foods to Avoid

There are not many foods to really avoid on a high-protein diet. Here are some guidelines:

- All pre-made baked goods such as cookies, bread, cake, granola bars, etc. Very few provide any protein at all, but they are definitely rich in unhealthy fats and sugar.
- Frozen entrées: most of them emphasize carbs at the expense of protein. Usually, you get a giant serving of rice with a few peas and carrot pieces in a pool of sugary sauce. Sometimes you can barely find the meat.
- Protein bars: you need to be really careful with these, as many will contain a high amount of sugar. The protein in these bars is also quite processed. Instead, try homemade fruit and nut bars.
- Unhealthy junk: chips, soda pop, candy and chocolate… even if some of them did offer minimal protein (chocolate for example) they are not worth the sugar and empty calories. Dark chocolate can be used in small amounts to add a rich flavour to protein-based baking.
- Deep-fried meat: it does contain protein, but it's covered with batter and then deep-fried in processed and unhealthy oils. Avoid if possible.

High Protein Baking

Almond Butter Crunch Granola Bar

Prep Time: 30 minutes

Servings: 8

INGREDIENTS

1 1/2 cup raw almonds

1 cup crunchy almond butter

1/4 cup flax seed (or chia seed)

1/2 cup dried pitted dates

2/3 cup shredded or flaked coconut

1/3 cup raw pumpkin seeds

1/2 teaspoon ground cinnamon

1/2 teaspoon vanilla

1 teaspoon Celtic sea salt

INSTRUCTIONS

1. Line loaf pan with parchment paper.
2. Add flax or chia to food processor or high-speed blender and process until finely ground, about 1 - 2 minutes.
3. Add 1 cup almonds and process until thick, smooth paste forms, up to 5 minutes.
4. Add dates and process until thick, fairly smooth mixture forms about 1 - 2 minutes. Transfer to medium mixing bowl.
5. Add remaining 1/2 cup almonds, almond butter, coconut, pumpkin seeds, cinnamon, vanilla, and salt. Stir to combine with large wooden spoon.

6. Transfer mixture to parchment lined pan and firmly press into bottom with hands or spatula. Place in refrigerator for 20 minutes.
7. Remove from refrigerator and cut into bars.
8. Serve chilled. Or allow to warm to room temperature and serve.

Vanilla Bean Shortbread Cookies

Prep Time: 5 minutes
Cook Time: 20 minutes
Servings: 12

INGREDIENTS

1 2/3 cups almond flour

2/3 cup almonds (blanched, skinless)

1/4 cup coconut oil (or cacao butter or coconut butter, melted)

1/4 cup date butter (or raw honey or agave)

1 Madagascar whole vanilla bean

1/4 teaspoon baking soda

1/4 teaspoon Celtic sea salt (plus extra)

INSTRUCTIONS
1. Preheat oven to 300 degrees F. Line sheet pan with parchment or baking mat.
2. Add almonds to food processor or high-speed blender and process until finely ground, about 2 minutes.
3. Add ground almonds to medium mixing bowl. Sift in almond flour, baking soda and salt.
4. Split vanilla bean pod in half and scrap insides into small mixing bowl. Add oil or melted butter and date butter. Mix to combine.
5. Pour vanilla mixture into flour mixture and mix to form dough.

6. Use mini ice cream scoop or tablespoon to drop portions of dough onto prepared sheet pan. Bake for 20 minutes, or until lightly browned.
7. Remove from oven and let cool at least 5 minutes.
8. Serve warm. Or let cool completely and serve room temperature.

Cranberry Pistachio Biscotti

Prep Time: 15 minutes

Cook Time: 45 minutes*

Servings: 6

INGREDIENTS

1 cup almond flour

1/2 cup coconut flour

1/2 cup raw honey (or date butter or agave)

1/4 cup pistachios

1/4 cup dried cranberries

1/2 teaspoon vanilla

1/2 teaspoon baking soda

1/4 teaspoon Celtic sea salt

INSTRUCTIONS

1. Preheat oven to 350 degrees F. Line sheet pan with parchment paper. Heat medium pan over medium heat.
2. In medium mixing bowl, blend almond flour, coconut flour, baking soda and salt with hand mixer or whisk.
3. Beat in honey and vanilla until well combined and thick, sticky dough forms. Mix in pistachios and cranberries with wooden spoon.
4. Form dough into flattened, uniform mound about 1 inch thick on sheet pan. Pat down mound to keep any nuts from sticking out.

5. Bake for about 15 minutes. Remove from oven and allow to cool for about 15 minutes.
6. Use a very sharp serrated knife to carefully cut biscotti log into 1/2 - 2/3 inch slices. Hold on to the mound and cut on a diagonal. If it becomes crumbly, stick it back together.
7. Lay slices on their sides and return to oven for 15 minutes.
8. *Turn oven off and leave oven door open a crack. Allow biscotti to cool and dry for at least 2 hours.
9. Serve room temperature.

Super-Protein Coconut Custard Pie

Prep Time: 10 minutes

Cook Time: 40 minutes

Servings: 12

INGREDIENTS

Crust

1 cup almond flour

1/4 cup almond butter (or cashew butter)

1/4 cup coconut oil (or cacao butter or ghee)

1 tablespoon raw honey (or agave or date butter)

1/4 teaspoon Celtic sea salt

Filling

2 cans (13 oz each) full-fat coconut milk

4 cage-free egg yolks

1 cup flaked coconut

1/2 cup nut milk

1/2 cup raw honey (or agave or date butter)

2 tablespoon tapioca flour

2 teaspoons vanilla

INSTRUCTIONS

1. Preheat oven to 350 degrees F. Lightly coat pie pan with coconut oil.

2. For *Crust*, add almond flour, almond butter, coconut oil, sweetener and salt to small mixing bowl, or food processor or high-speed blender. Mix or process until dough forms.
3. Firmly press dough into pie pan with hands.
4. For *Filling*, add coconut milk, flaked coconut, egg yolks, nut milk, sweetener, tapioca flour and vanilla to medium mixing bowl, or clean food processor or high-speed blender. Mix or process to combine.
5. Pour *Filling* into *Crust* and bake for 40 - 50 minutes, until set and golden brown.
6. Remove from oven and let cool at least 30 minutes.
7. Slice and serve room temperature. Or refrigerate at least 30 minutes and serve chilled.

Vanilla Peach Cake

Prep Time: 10 minutes

Cook Time: 50 minutes

Servings: 12

INGREDIENTS

4 ripe peaches

3/4 cup coconut flour

10 cage-free eggs

1/2 cup coconut oil (or cacao or coconut butter)

1/3 cup raw honey (or agave, date butter or stevia)

2 tablespoons tapioca flour (or arrowroot powder)

1 teaspoon baking soda

1 1/2 teaspoons vanilla

1 teaspoon Celtic sea salt

INSTRUCTIONS

1. Preheat oven to 350 degrees F. Line square or rectangular baking dish with parchment paper, or coat with coconut oil.
2. Slice peaches in half, twist to release from pit and remove pit. Dice 2 peaches and set aside.
3. Roughly chop remaining peaches and add to food processor or high-speed blender. Process until almost smooth, about 1 minute.
4. Add eggs, oil or butter, and flour to processor in 2 batches. Process until well combined, about 1 - 2 minutes. Add sweetener, baking

soda, vanilla and salt. Process until light, thick batter forms. Stir in diced peaches.

5. Pour batter into prepared baking pan and bake about 50 minutes, until golden brown and toothpick inserted into center comes out moist but clean.
6. Remove from oven and let cool about 10 minutes.
7. Slice and serve warm. Or let cool completely and serve room temperature or warm.

Walnut Raisin Cookies

Prep Time: 10 minutes

Cook Time: 15 minutes

Servings: 12

INGREDIENTS

1 1/4 cups almond flour

1 cage-free egg

1/4 cup coconut oil (or cacao or coconut butter)

1/4 cup raw honey (or agave or date butter)

1/4 cup cashew butter

1/2 cup walnuts

1/4 cup raisins

1 teaspoon baking powder

1 teaspoon vanilla

1/4 teaspoon Celtic sea salt

INSTRUCTIONS

1. Preheat oven to 350 degrees F. Line sheet pan with parchment or baking mat.
2. Sift flour, baking powder and salt into medium mixing bowl. Beat with whisk or hand mixer to lighten. Add egg, oil or butter, sweetener, cashew butter, vanilla and salt. Mix well to form dough.
3. Chop walnuts and add to bowl with raisins. Mix to combine.

4. Shape dough into 12 balls and place onto prepared baking sheet. Flatten slightly with hand or spatula.
5. Place in oven and bake 10 - 15 minutes, until golden brown along edges.
6. Remove from oven and let cool 5 minutes.
7. Serve warm. Or transfer to wire rack to cool completely and serve room temperature.

Indian Sweet Almond Fudge

Prep Time: 15 minutes*

Cook Time: 30 minutes

Servings: 6

INGREDIENTS

1 cup blanched almonds (skinless)

1 cup nut milk

1/4 cup ghee (or cacao or coconut butter)

1/4 - 1/2 cup date butter (or raw honey or agave)

1/4 teaspoon ground cardamom (optional)

1/4 teaspoon ground ginger (optional)

Pinch saffron (optional)

INSTRUCTIONS

1. Heat medium pan over medium heat. Add 2 tablespoon ghee or butter.
2. Add almonds and nut milk to food processor or high-speed blender. Process until finely ground, about 2 minutes.
3. Add almond mixture to hot oiled pan and cook about 5 minutes, stirring constantly with large wooden spoon. Mixture may stick to pan, but do not let burn.
4. Add sweetener and bring to a simmer, about 5 - 10 minutes. Continue to stir constantly. Add remaining ghee or butter and optional spices.

5. Stir until mixture turn golden and pulls together, about 10 minutes. Transfer to serving dish.
6. Serve warm. Or let cool completely and serve room temperature.

Asian Sesame Cookies

Prep Time: 10 minutes

Cook Time: 20 minutes

Servings: 12

INGREDIENTS

1 1/2 cups almond flour

1 cage-free egg

1/2 cup date butter (or raw honey or agave)

1/2 cup coconut oil (or cacao or coconut butter, melted)

1 cup sesame seeds

3/4 cup flaked or shredded coconut

1 teaspoon baking powder

1 teaspoon baking soda

1/2 teaspoon vanilla

1/2 teaspoon Celtic sea salt

INSTRUCTIONS

1. Preheat oven to 350 degrees F. Heat medium pan over medium heat. Line sheet pan with parchment paper or baking mat.
2. Add sesame seeds and coconut to hot dry pan. Toast 5 - 10 minutes, until lightly golden. Remove from pan and set aside.
3. Add egg, sweetener, oil or butter, and vanilla to small mixing bowl. Mix well with wooden spoon or hand mixer. Add toasted sesame seeds and coconut and mix well.

4. In medium mixing bowl, sift together flour, baking powder, baking soda and salt. Add egg mixture to flour mixture and mix well until dough forms.
5. Form dough into 1 inch balls and place on prepared sheet pan. Flatten with fork and bake 10 - 15 minutes, until golden brown and cooked through.
6. Remove from oven and transfer to wire racks to cool completely.
7. Serve room temperature.

Blueberry Scones

Prep Time: 5 minutes

Cook Time: 25 minutes

Servings: 8

INGREDIENTS

2 cups almond flour

1/3 cup arrowroot powder (or tapioca flour)

1 cage-free egg

1/2 cup dried or frozen blueberries

1/4 cup coconut oil

2 tablespoons sweetener*

2 teaspoons baking powder

1/2 teaspoon vanilla

1/2 teaspoon sea salt

1/4 teaspoon ground cinnamon (optional)

INSTRUCTIONS

1. Preheat oven to 350 degrees F. Line sheet pan with parchment or coat with coconut oil.
2. Whisk together almond flour, arrowroot powder, baking powder, salt, vanilla and cinnamon (optional) in medium mixing bowl.
3. In small mixing bowl, beat egg, oil and sweetener with hand mixer or whisk. Add egg mixture to dry ingredients and mix until well combined.

4. Fold in blueberries. Form dough into ball and place on sheet pan. Pat down to flatten to about 1/2 inch thick circle.
5. Cut into eight wedges with pizza cutter or sharp knife. Arrange at least 1 inch apart on sheet pan and bake for 20 - 25 minutes, or until edges are golden brown.
6. Remove from oven and let cool at least 10 minutes.
7. Serve room temperature.

Classic Bagels

Prep Time: 10 minutes

Cook Time: 25 minutes

Servings: 8

INGREDIENTS

2 cups almond flour

2 tablespoons coconut flour

2 tablespoons ground chia seed (or flax meal)

1 tablespoon tapioca flour (or arrowroot powder)

4 cage-free eggs

1/3 cup apple cider vinegar

2 tablespoons unsweetened applesauce

2 tablespoons sweetener*

1 teaspoon baking soda

1/2 teaspoon sea salt

INSTRUCTIONS
1. Preheat oven to 350 degrees. Lightly coat donut pan with coconut oil.
2. Add almond, coconut and tapioca flours, chia meal, baking soda and salt to food processor or bullet blender, and process for 1 minute.
3. Add eggs, sweetener, applesauce and apple cider vinegar to flour mixture and process until fully blended, about 1 - 2 minutes.
4. Carefully scoop batter into donut pan, avoiding raised middle.

5. Place in oven and bake about 20 - 25 minutes.
6. Remove and let cool about 5 minutes. Then remove from pan.
7. Slice in half and serve immediately. Or let cool completely and serve room temperature.

NOTE: Bake in 8 round mini cake pans lightly coated with coconut oil if you do not have a donut pan.

stevia, raw honey or agave nectar

Avocado Club Muffin

Prep Time: 10 minutes

Cook Time: 15 minutes

Servings: 12

INGREDIENTS

1 cup almond flour

2 cage-free eggs

1 avocado

4 slices nitrate-free bacon

1 tablespoon sweetener*

1 teaspoon apple cider vinegar

1 teaspoon baking powder

1/4 teaspoon ground white pepper (or black pepper)

INSTRUCTIONS

1. Preheat oven to 350 degrees F. Line muffin pan with paper liners or light coat with coconut oil. Heat medium pan over medium-high heat.
2. Finely chop bacon and add to hot pan. Sauté until crisp and cooked through, about 5 minutes. Set aside.
3. Beat eggs, sweetener and vinegar in medium mixing bowl with hand mixer or whisk until thick and slightly foamy.
4. Slice avocado in half. Scoop flesh of one half into egg mixture. Add bacon and drippings, almond flour, baking powder and black pepper and mix until combined.

5. Dice remaining avocado flesh and fold into batter.
6. Use ice cream scoop or tablespoon to scoop batter into prepared muffin pan.
7. Bake about 15 - 20 minutes, until edges are golden brown and tops are firm.
8. Remove from oven and let cool for 5 minutes.
9. Serve warm. Or cool completely and serve temperature.

NOTE: Bake in square oiled baking pan for 30 - 35 minutes for **Avocado Club Bread**.

stevia, raw honey or agave nectar

Carrot Cake Cookie Bars

Prep Time: 10 minutes

Cook Time: 25 minutes

Servings: 12

INGREDIENTS

2 cups almond meal

2 cups shredded carrots (about 4 large carrots)

3 cage-free eggs

1/4 cup coconut oil

1/2 cup unsweetened applesauce

1/2 cup flaked coconut

1/4 cup sweetener*

2 teaspoons vanilla

2 teaspoons ground cinnamon

1 teaspoon ground nutmeg

1/2 teaspoon ground black pepper

1/2 teaspoon sea salt

INSTRUCTIONS

1. Preheat oven to 350 Degrees F. Line baking pan with parchment or coat lightly with coconut oil.
2. Grate carrots, or process in food processor or bullet blender until finely chopped. Add to medium bowl.
3. Add eggs, oil, applesauce and sweetener to food processor or bullet blender. Process until thickened and light, about 1 - 2 minutes.

4. Pour egg mixture into carrots. Sift in almond flour and salt. Add vanilla and spices. Mix well with a wooden spoon or hand mixer. Stir in coconut.
5. Press dough evenly into prepared baking pan and bake about 25 minutes, or until firm and golden brown.
6. Remove from oven and allow to cool about 10 minutes.
7. Slice into bars and serve warm. Or let cool completely and serve room temperature.

stevia, raw honey, agave nectar or maple syrup

Ginger Spice Cookies

Prep Time: 15 minutes

Cook Time: 15 minutes

Servings: 6

INGREDIENTS

1 1/2 cups almond flour

1 cage-free egg

1/4 cup sweetener*

2 tablespoons coconut oil

1 teaspoon ground chia seed (or flax meal)

1/4 teaspoon baking soda

1 tablespoon ground ginger

1/2 teaspoon ground clove

Pinch all spice

Pinch ground black pepper

Pinch sea salt

INSTRUCTIONS

1. Preheat oven to 350 degrees F. Line sheet pan with parchment or baking mat, or lightly coat with coconut oil.
2. Beat egg, oil, sweetener and chia meal in medium mixing bowl with hand mixer or whisk.
3. Add almond flour, baking soda, salt and spices. Mix until combined.
4. Chill batter in freezer for 5 - 10 minutes.

5. Scoop chilled batter into 6 large rounds on prepared sheet pan. Press into disk shape with hand.
6. Bake for about 15 minutes, until firm around the edges and golden brown.
7. Remove from oven and let cool about 10 minutes.
8. Serve warm. Or let cool completely and serve room temperature.

raw honey, agave nectar, grade B maple syrup, molasses

Rosemary Basil Scones

Prep Time: 10 minutes

Cook Time: 25 minutes

Servings: 8

INGREDIENTS

2 cups almond flour

1/3 cup arrowroot flour

1 egg

1/4 cup organic coconut oil

1/2 lemon

2 tablespoons sweetener*

2 teaspoons baking powder

2 sprigs fresh rosemary

5 - 6 large basil leaves (or 1 1/2 teaspoons dried basil)

1/2 teaspoon vanilla

1/2 teaspoon sea salt

1/4 cup hazelnuts (optional)

INSTRUCTIONS

1. Preheat oven to 350 degrees F. Line sheet pan with parchment or coat with coconut oil.
2. Whisk together flours, baking powder, salt and vanilla in large mixing bowl.
3. Zest 1/2 lemon into small mixing bowl. Finely chop rosemary and chiffon fresh basil. Add herbs to bowl with egg and sweetener.

Beat with hand mixer or whisk while slowly pouring in coconut oil.
4. Add egg mixture to flour blend and mix until well combined.
5. Chop and fold in hazelnuts (optional). Form dough into ball and place on sheet pan. Flatten to 1/2 inch thick circle with hands.
6. Cut into eight wedges with pizza cutter or sharp knife. Arrange at least 1 inch apart on sheet pan and bake for 20 - 25 minutes , or until edges are golden brown.
7. Remove and let cool. Serve room temperature.

orange juice, raw honey, agave nectar or maple syrup

Cinnamon Cashew Rugalach

Prep Time: 25 minutes

Cook Time: 20 minutes

Servings: 12

INSTRUCTIONS

Crust

2 cups almond flour

2 eggs

2 tablespoons coconut oil

2 tablespoons cacao butter (or full-fat coconut milk)

2 tablespoons sweetener*

1 teaspoon baking powder

1/2 teaspoon baking soda

1/2 teaspoon vanilla

1/4 teaspoon ground cinnamon

1/4 teaspoon sea salt

Filling

1 cup cashews

1/4 cup dried pitted dates

1/2 cup water

2 tablespoons sweetener*

2 teaspoons ground cinnamon

1/2 teaspoon vanilla

INSTRUCTIONS

1. For *Crust*, sift almond flour into medium mixing bowl. Add baking soda and powder, vanilla, cinnamon and salt.
2. Whisk eggs and sweetener in small mixing bowl, then add to flour mixture and combine. Slowly add coconut oil and cacao butter or coconut milk until malleable dough comes together.
3. Roll in plastic wrap or wrap tightly in parchment and refrigerate for 15 minutes.
4. Preheat oven to 350 degrees F. Line sheet pan with parchment or baking mat. Cover cutting board with parchment. Heat medium pot over medium-high heat.
5. For *Filling*, bring 1/2 cup water, dates, cinnamon and vanilla to boil In small pot. Reduce heat and simmer until reduced and most liquid evaporates, about 5 minutes.
6. Add cashews to food processor or bullet blender. Process to chop cashews. Add dates and sweetener to cashews and process until dates break down and sandy mixture forms.
7. Remove dough from refrigerator. Roll dough out on parchment covered cutting board to about 1/8 inch thick rectangle with rolling pin.
8. Spread *Filling* over dough. Use sharp knife or pizza cutter to cut dough into 12 rectangles.
9. Roll up dough pieces and arrange on prepared sheet pan. Place in oven and bake 15 - 20 minutes, or until dough is golden brown and cooked through.
10. Remove from oven and allow to cool about 5 minutes.
11. Serve immediately. Or allow to cool completely and serve room temperature.

*stevia, raw honey or agave nectar

Kefir Sourdough Rolls

Prep Time: 10 minutes*

Cook Time: 20 minutes

Servings: 8

INGREDIENTS

Starter

1 1/3 cups drained kefir milk (no kefir grains left)

1/2 cup almond flour

1/4 cup tapioca flour (or arrowroot powder)

1/2 cup warm water

2 tablespoons sweetener*

Rolls

1/2 cup almond flour

1/2 cup coconut flour

1/4 cup coconut oil

1/2 cup warm water

1 tablespoon apple cider vinegar

1 teaspoon baking soda

1 teaspoon sea salt

INSTRUCTIONS

1. *For *Starter*, add 1/2 cup water to small pot and heat over medium heat until warm. Add all *Starter* ingredients to medium mixing

bowl and mix together. Cover tightly with aluminum foil or parchment paper. Store in a warm area for 12 - 18 hours.
2. Preheat oven to 350 degrees F. Line sheet pan with parchment paper or coat with coconut oil. Or coat muffin pan with coconut oil.
3. For *Rolls*, add 1/2 cup water to small pot and heat over medium heat until warm. Sift almond flour, coconut flour, baking soda and salt into Starter. Add coconut oil and vinegar and mix to combine. Add enough warm water to form sticky dough.
4. Shape dough into rolls with hands and place on prepared sheet pan, or scoop into muffin pan.
5. Place in oven for 15 - 20 minute, until golden brown and cooked through.
6. Remove from oven and serve warm. Or allow to cool completely and serve room temperature.

* raw honey or agave nectar

Chocolate Pecan Shortbread Cookies

Prep Time: 5 minutes
Cook Time: 20 minutes
Servings: 12

INGREDIENTS

1 1/2 cups almond flour

1 1/2 cup pecans

1/4 cup cocoa powder

1/4 cup coconut oil (or melted cacao butter)

1/4 cup sweetener*

1 teaspoons vanilla

1/4 teaspoon baking soda

1/2 teaspoon sea salt

INSTRUCTIONS

1. Preheat oven to 300 degrees F. Line sheet pan with parchment or baking mat.
2. Add 1 cup pecans to food processor or high-speed blender and process until finely ground.
3. Add ground pecans to medium mixing bowl. Sift in almond flour, cocoa, baking soda and salt.
4. Chop remaining pecans and add to small mixing bowl. Add coconut oil or melted cacao butter, sweetener and vanilla to pecans. Mix to combine.
5. Pour wet mixture into dry ingredients and mix to form dough.

6. Use mini ice cream scoop or tablespoon to drop portions of dough onto prepared sheet pan.
7. Place in oven and bake 20 minutes, or until lightly browned.
8. Remove from oven and let cool at least 5 minutes.
9. Let cool completely and serve room temperature. Or serve warm.

raw honey, agave nectar or maple syrup

Cocoa Gingerbread

Prep Time: 5 minutes

Cook Time: 20 minutes

Servings: 8

INGREDIENTS

2 cups almond flour

2 tablespoons ground chia seed (or flax meal)

2 eggs

1/2 cup unsweetened applesauce

1/4 cup coconut oil

1/4 cup sweetener*

1/4 cup cocoa powder

1 tablespoon baking powder

1 teaspoon baking soda

2 tablespoons ground ginger

1 tablespoon ground cinnamon

1 teaspoon ground black pepper

1 teaspoon vanilla

1/2 teaspoon ground cloves

2 oz fresh ginger juice (optional)

INSTRUCTIONS

1. Preheat oven to 350 degrees F. Coat 2 small loaf pans with coconut oil.

2. Beat eggs in large mixing bowl with hand mixer or whisk until light and thickened, about 2 minutes. Add applesauce, oil, sweetener and ginger juice (optional). Beat well.
3. Sift all dry ingredients Into medium mixing bowl. Slowly beat flour mixture into egg mixture.
4. Pour batter into prepared loaf pans and bake for 20 - 25 minutes, or until toothpick inserted into center comes out clean.
5. Let cool at least 5 minutes. Insert knife around edges and remove brad from pan.
6. Slice and serve warm. Or let cool completely and serve room temperature.

NOTE: Bake in large oiled loaf pan for 35 - 45 minutes for **Cocoa Gingerbread Loaf**.

raw honey, agave nectar, maple syrup, molasses

State Fair Fry Bread

Prep Time: 5 minutes

Cook Time: 15 minutes

Servings: 2

INGREDIENTS

1 cup coconut flour

1 cup almond flour (or cashew flour)

1/4 cup tapioca flour/starch

3 eggs

1/2 cup coconut oil

1/2 cup full-fat coconut milk

1 teaspoon baking powder

2 tablespoons sweetener*

Pinch sea salt

Water (for thinning)

Coconut oil (for cooking)

INSTRUCTIONS
1. Heat medium skillet over medium-high heat and coat generously with coconut oil.
2. Blend eggs, oil, milk and sweetener in food processor or bullet blender until smooth and a bit airy.

3. In medium bowl, combine flours, baking powder and salt. Add egg mixture and combine to form soft dough. If too tough, add water 1 tablespoon at a time.
4. Form dough into 2 large flat rounds with hands. Place 1 round in pan and cook about 3 minutes, or until puffed and browned. Flip fry bread with tongs or spatula and cook another 3 minutes, or until golden and cooked through.
5. Repeat with remaining dough. Re-oil pan as necessary.
6. Drain hot fry bread on paper towel. Serve warm.

NOTE: For **Baked Fry Bread** , generously coat two 9-inch round cake pans with coconut oil. Press dough into pans and brush tops with coconut oil. Bake at 425 degrees F in for 15 minutes, or until cooked through and golden.

stevia, raw honey or agave nectar

Easy Biscuits

Prep Time: 5 minutes
Cook Time: 15 minutes
Servings: 8

INGREDIENTS

2 1/2 cups fine ground almond flour

2 eggs

1/4 cup coconut oil

1 teaspoon baking soda

1/2 teaspoon sea salt

1 tablespoon sweetener*

INSTRUCTIONS

1. Preheat oven to 350 degrees F. Line sheet pan with parchment paper.
2. Combine almond flour, baking soda and salt in medium bowl.
3. Separate egg whites into separate medium bowl, and yolk into small bowl. Beat egg whites to soft peaks with hand mixer or whisk.
4. Mix yolks, oil and sweetener into whites. Mix wet ingredients into dry to form soft, solid dough.
5. Roll dough into eight (8) 1-inch thick round biscuits with hands. Place on parchment covered sheet pan and bake for 12 - 15 minutes, or until golden and firm on top. Serve warm.

NOTE: Oil square baking pan, gently press in dough, cut into 9 squares, and bake for 20 - 25 minutes for break-away pan biscuits.

stevia, raw honey or agave nectar

Cranberry Pistachio Scones

Prep Time: 10 minutes
Cook Time: 25 minutes
Servings: 8

INGREDIENTS

2 cups almond flour

1/3 cup arrowroot flour

1 egg

1/4 cup organic coconut oil

2 tablespoons liquid sweetener*

2 teaspoons baking powder

1/2 teaspoon vanilla

1/2 teaspoon sea salt

1/4 cup pistachio nuts

1/4 cup dried cranberries

INSTRUCTIONS

1. Preheat oven to 350 degrees F. Line sheet pan with parchment or coat with coconut oil.
2. Whisk together flours, baking powder, salt and vanilla in large mixing bowl.
3. In small mixing bowl, combine egg, oil and sweetener with hand mixer or whisk. Beat briskly while slowly pouring in coconut oil.
4. Add egg mixture to flour blend and mix until well combined.

5. Fold in cranberries and pistachios until incorporated. Form dough into ball and place on sheet pan. Pat down to flatten to about 1/2 inch thick circle.
6. Cut into eight wedges with pizza cutter or sharp knife. Arrange at least 1 inch apart on sheet pan and bake for 20 - 25 minutes, or until edges are golden brown.
7. Remove and cool. Serve room temperature.

fresh squeezed orange juice, raw honey, agave nectar or grade B maple syrup

Avocado Spice Bread

Prep Time: 5 minutes

Cook Time: 20 minutes

Servings: 12

INGREDIENTS

1 3/4 cups almond flour

1/4 cup flax seed meal (or ground chia seed)

3 eggs

3 avocados

1/2 cup unsweetened applesauce (or apple butter)

1/4 cup sweetener*

1/2 cup fresh squeezed orange juice

1 tablespoon orange zest

1 tablespoon baking powder

1 teaspoon ground cinnamon

1 teaspoon ground allspice

1 teaspoon ground black pepper

1 teaspoon sea salt

INSTRUCTIONS

1. Preheat oven to 350 degrees F. Coat square baking pan with coconut oil.
2. Slice avocados in half, pit, and scoop flesh into food processor or blender. Add eggs, applesauce, sweetener and orange juice and blend until smooth.

3. Pour avocado blend into medium mixing bowl. Stir in almond flour, flax meal, baking powder, salt, orange zest and spices until combined.
4. Pour batter into oiled baking pan. Bake 20 - 25 minutes, or until firm but springy in center.
5. Serve warm or room temperature.

NOTE: Bake in lined or oiled muffin pan for 15 - 20 minutes for **Avocado Spice Muffins**.

stevia, raw honey or agave nectar

Apple Upside Down Cakes

Prep Time: 5 minutes

Cook Time: 15 minutes

Servings: 2

INGREDIENTS

1 3/4 cups almond meal

2 eggs

3/4 cup almond milk

2 tablespoons sweetener*

1 teaspoon baking powder

Juice of 1/2 lemon

1 teaspoon vanilla

1 teaspoon ground cinnamon

1 teaspoon ground nutmeg

1/4 teaspoon salt

1 tart apple

1/2 cup crushed pecans

INSTRUCTIONS

1. Heat large skillet over medium-high heat and lightly coat with coconut oil.
2. In medium bowl combine lemon juice, vanilla, cinnamon and nutmeg.
3. Peel and core apple, then slice in half length-wise. Lay halves down on flat side and slice thinly from top of apple to bottom.

Carefully toss apple slices in lemon juice and spices. Try not to break any.
4. Arrange apple slices into a circle by overlapping at the bottom and fanning out. Try to make at least 4 circles.
5. Add eggs and almond milk into leftover lemon juice and spices and whisk until combined. Add almond flour, salt and baking powder. Whisk until smooth.
6. Use oiled spatula to lift apples, keeping their arrangement, and place into hot pan. Get at least two apple arrangements into pan together. Sprinkle chopped pecans into pan around apple circles.
7. Use ladle or dry measure cup to pour 1/3 cup of batter over and around apple arrangements in skillet. Do not let pancakes touch as they spread.
8. Cook until sides of pancakes are firm and batter bubbles up a bit. About 3 - 4 minutes.
9. Flip pancakes with spatula, careful not to disturb apples. Cook for additional minute, or until cooked through. Repeat with remaining batter. Re-oil pan if necessary.
10. Pancakes will be slightly delicate, so flip and plate with care.
11. Sprinkle with cinnamon. Serve warm.

stevia, raw honey, or agave nectar

Cashew Belgian Waffles

Prep Time: 10 minutes

Cook Time: 10 minutes

Servings: 2

INGREDIENTS

Waffles:

1 cup cashew flour (or finely ground raw cashews)

1/4 coconut flour

3 eggs, separated

1/4 cup coconut oil

4 tablespoons sweetener

1 tablespoon aluminum-free baking soda

1 teaspoon vanilla

1 pinch sea salt

1 teaspoon ground cinnamon (optional)

Topping:

1 cup fresh fruit

1/2 teaspoon vanilla

2 tablespoons water

1 tablespoon sweetener*

DIRECTIONS

1. Preheat waffle iron. Use wadded paper towel to carefully coat with coconut oil.

2. Combine flours, salt and baking soda in small bowl. In large bowl, whisk together egg yolks, oil, vanilla, plus sweetener and cinnamon (optional).
3. In separate bowl, beat egg whites to medium-stiff peaks with hand mixer. Stir flour mixture into the egg yolk mixture. Gently fold egg whites into batter.
4. Pour portion of batter onto hot waffle iron. Cook 4 - 5 minutes, until golden brown and crisp. Repeat with remain batter
5. While waffles are cooking, combine all **Topping** ingredients in small pan. Cook over stovetop until reduced and thick.
6. Top waffles with fruit compote or agave syrup (optional). Serve hot.

stevia, raw honey, or agave nectar

Fruit And Nut Cake

Prep Time: 10 minutes

Cook Time: 25 minutes

Servings: 8

INGREDIENTS

1 1/2 cup almond flour

4 eggs

2 tablespoons coconut oil

Juice of orange half

1/4 cup sweetener*

1/2 cup walnuts

1/4 cup pecans

1/2 cup dried pitted dates

1/2 cup dried cherries

1/4 cup dried apricots

1/4 cup raisins

1/2 teaspoon baking soda

1 teaspoon ground ginger

1 teaspoon vanilla

1/2 teaspoon sea salt

Zest of orange half

INSTRUCTIONS

1. Preheat oven to 350 degrees F. Lightly coat 2 small loaf pans or one Bundt pan with coconut oil.

2. Sift almond flour, baking soda and salt into large mixing bowl.
3. Chop walnuts, pecans, apricots and dates. Then stir all dried fruit and nuts into flour mixture.
4. In medium mixing bowl, mix eggs, coconut oil, juice and zest of half an orange, sweetener, ginger and vanilla. Then pour and mix into dry ingredients until just combined.
5. Scoop batter into loaf pans or Bundt pan, and smooth tops with spatula.
6. Bake 20 - 30 minutes, or until firm, browned and firm in the center.
7. Remove from oven and allow to cool before slicing.
8. Serve warm or room temperature.

stevia, raw honey or agave nectar

Chocolate Almond Biscotti

Prep Time: 15 minutes

Cook Time: 35* minutes

Servings: 6

INGREDIENTS

1 cup almond flour

1/2 cup coconut flour

1/2 cup sweetener*

1/3 cup almonds

2 tablespoons cocoa powder

1 teaspoon vanilla

1/2 teaspoon baking soda

1/4 teaspoon sea salt

INSTRUCTIONS

1. Preheat oven to 350 degrees F. Line sheet pan with parchment paper. Heat medium pan over medium heat.
2. Add almonds to hot dry pan and toast for about 5 minutes, until aromatic. Stir frequently. Remove from heat and set aside.
3. In medium mixing bowl, blend almond flour, coconut flour, cocoa powder, baking soda and salt with hand mixer or whisk.
4. Beat in sweetener and vanilla until well combined and thick, sticky dough forms. Mix in toasted almonds with wooden spoon.
5. Form dough into flattened, uniform mound about 1 inch thick on sheet pan. Pat down mound to keep any almonds from sticking out.

6. Bake for about 15 minutes . Remove and allow to cool for about 15 minutes.
7. Use a very sharp serrated knife to carefully cut biscotti log into 1/2 - 2/3 inch slices. Hold onto the mound and cut on a diagonal. If it becomes crumbly, stick it back together.
8. Lace slice on sides and return to oven for 15 minutes.
9. Try to cut so that you're holding on to the edges of the log to keep it from crumbling. If parts come apart, you can stick them back together as the mixture is still kind of sticky.
10. Lay the biscotti flat and return to oven for 15 minutes.
11. *Turn oven off and leave oven door open a crack. Allow the biscotti to cool and dry for at least 2 hours.
12. Serve room temperature.

raw honey, agave nectar, maple syrup, or any combination

Wild Mince Meat Pie

Prep Time: 20 minutes

Cook Time: 30 minutes

Servings: 8

INGREDIENTS

Crust

4 cups almond flour

2 eggs

1/4 cup coconut oil

1/2 teaspoon sea salt

Filling

12 oz grass-fed beef

2 sweet apples

2 tart apples

1 cup beef stock

1/4 cup sweetener*

Juice of 1 orange

Zest of 1 orange

1/4 cup arrowroot powder

1/4 cup apple cider vinegar

1 cup raisins

1/2 cup dried pitted dates

1/2 cup dried pitted prunes

1/2 cup dried cherries

2 teaspoons ground cinnamon

1 teaspoon ground nutmeg

1/2 teaspoon ground cloves

1/2 teaspoon ground black pepper

1/2 teaspoon salt

INSTRUCTIONS

1. Preheat oven to 350 degrees F. Heat large pot over medium-high heat and lightly coat with coconut oil. Lightly oil pie plate. Prepare 4 sheets of parchment.
2. Place beef in hot oiled pan and brown on each side for about 5 - 7 minutes, until just cooked through. Remove beef and set aside. Add beef stock to pot.
3. Mix all *Crust* ingredients together in medium bowl until dough forms. Divide dough in half and use rolling pin to roll dough between two parchment sheets into circles to fit about 1 inch over pie plate.
4. Press one dough circle into pie plate. Crimp edges to create small lip. Bake for 5 minutes, then remove and set aside.
5. Peel, core and grate or dice apples. Add to beef stock with sweetener, zest and juice of orange, vinegar, raisins, cherries, spices and salt. Dice beef, prunes and dates, and add to pot. Stir in arrowroot powder and thicken for a few minutes.
6. Once mixture comes together pour into par baked pie shell. Top with second dough sheet and crimp edges to fit into bottom crust.
7. Use sharp knife to slice top crust a few times for venting.
8. Bake pie for 30 minutes, or until crust is golden brown.
9. Remove from oven and allow to cool for about 20 minutes.

10. Slice and serve warm. Or allow to cool completely and serve room temperature.

stevia, raw honey or agave nectar

High-Protein Pretzel Sticks

Prep Time: 15 minutes

Cook Time: 20 minutes

Servings: 12

INGREDIENTS

1 1/2 cups almond flour

3 tablespoons coconut flour

3 cage-free eggs

2 tablespoons ghee (or cacao butter or coconut oil, melted)

2 tablespoons Celtic sea salt

1 teaspoon water

INSTRUCTIONS

1. Beat 2 eggs in small mixing bowl with hand mixer to whisk. Set aside.
2. In medium bowl, sift almond flour, 1/2 teaspoon salt, and butter or oil. Mix to combine.
3. Add beaten eggs and 1 tablespoon coconut flour. Mix well. Let mixture sit 1 minute, then add second tablespoon of coconut flour. Blend again and let sit another minute. Add last tablespoon of coconut flour. Mix and set aside 5 minutes.
4. Preheat oven to 350 degrees F. Line sheet pan with parchment or baking mat.

5. Take portion of dough about the size of a golf ball and roll into long, thin log. Place on prepared sheet pan. Repeat with remaining dough.
6. Place pan in oven and bake 10 minutes.
7. Beat remaining egg in small bowl with 1 teaspoon water.
8. Remove pan from oven. Increase oven temperature to 400 degrees F.
9. Lightly brush tops of pretzels with the egg wash and sprinkle with generously with remaining salt.
10. Once oven is preheated, return pan to oven and bake 5 minutes.
11. Remove from oven and let cool slightly.
12. Serve warm. Or cool completely and serve room temperature.

Slow Cooker Berry Cobbler

Prep Time: 10 minutes

Cook Time: 4 hours

Servings: 6

INGREDIENTS

Filling

1 pint strawberries (fresh or thawed)

1 1/4 cup blueberries (fresh or frozen)

1 1/4 cup raspberries (fresh or frozen)

1/4 cup raw honey (or stevia, agave or date butter)

2 tablespoons tapioca flour (or arrowroot powder)

1/2 teaspoon ground cinnamon

Topping

1 cup almond flour

1/2 cup almonds

1/2 cup full-fat coconut milk

1/4 cup cacao butter (or coconut butter or coconut oil, chilled)

1/4 cup dried pitted dates

1/2 teaspoon baking powder

1/2 teaspoon cinnamon

1/2 teaspoon vanilla

INSTRUCTIONS

1. Cut tops off strawberries and roughly chop. Add to large mixing bowl with blueberries, raspberries, honey, tapioca flour and cinnamon. Toss to coat well. Transfer to slow cooker.
2. Add almonds and pitted dates to food processor or high-speed blender. Process until finely chopped, about 30 seconds. Add almond flour, chilled butter or oil, coconut milk, baking powder, cinnamon and vanilla. Pulse until crumbly dough comes together, about 1 minute.
3. Drop spoonfuls of dough over fruit mixture. Cover slow cooker with tea towel, then with lid. Turn on to high and cook 3 - 4 hours until, the topping has browned and crisped and fruit is bubbling.
4. Turn off slow cooker and carefully remove lid. Use large serving spoon to transfer to serving dish.
5. Serve warm.

Avocado Club Muffin

Prep Time: 10 minutes
Cook Time: 15 minutes
Servings: 12

INGREDIENTS

1 cup almond flour
2 cage-free eggs
1 avocado
4 slices nitrate-free bacon
1 tablespoon sweetener*
1 teaspoon apple cider vinegar
1 teaspoon baking powder
1/4 teaspoon ground white pepper (or black pepper)

INSTRUCTIONS

1. Preheat oven to 350 degrees F. Line muffin pan with paper liners or light coat with coconut oil. Heat medium pan over medium-high heat.
2. Finely chop bacon and add to hot pan. Sauté until crisp and cooked through, about 5 minutes. Set aside.
3. Beat eggs, sweetener and vinegar in medium mixing bowl with hand mixer or whisk until thick and slightly foamy.
4. Slice avocado in half. Scoop flesh of one half into egg mixture. Add bacon and drippings, almond flour, baking powder and black pepper and mix until combined.

5. Dice remaining avocado flesh and fold into batter.
6. Use ice cream scoop or tablespoon to scoop batter into prepared muffin pan.
7. Bake about 15 - 20 minutes, until edges are golden brown and tops are firm.
8. Remove from oven and let cool for 5 minutes.
9. Serve warm. Or cool completely and serve temperature.

NOTE: Bake in square oiled baking pan for 30 - 35 minutes for **Avocado Club Bread**.

stevia, raw honey or agave nectar

High Protein Dinners

High Protein Chicken Satay

Prep Time: 10 minutes*

Cook Time: 25 minutes

Servings: 4

INGREDIENTS

16 oz (1 lb) boneless skinless chicken

12 wooden skewers (soaked in water for 1 hour)

Marinade

1 tablespoon pure fish sauce (or liquid aminos or coconut Aminos)

2 inch piece fresh ginger root

1 garlic clove

Satay Sauce

13 oz (1 can) full-fat coconut milk

1/2 cup crunchy almond butter

1 tablespoon raw honey or agave nectar

1 tablespoon pure fish sauce (or tamari or coconut aminos)

1 teaspoon apple cider vinegar (or liquid aminos or coconut vinegar)

4 shallots

2 garlic cloves

2 inch piece fresh ginger root

2 small red chili peppers

1 1/2 tablespoons lime juice

Coconut oil (for cooking)

INSTRUCTIONS

1. *Cut chicken into 1 inch strips. For *Marinade*, peel and mince garlic and ginger. Add to medium mixing bowl with fish sauce and whisk. Add chicken and toss with until coated. Cover and set aside to marinate for 1 hour.
2. *Soak wooden skewers in water in shallow dish for 1 hour.
3. Heat medium pan or wok over medium heat and add 1 tablespoon coconut oil.
4. For *Satay Sauce*, peel and mince shallots, garlic and ginger. Slice peppers. Add to hot pan and sauté until softened, about 5 - 8 minutes.
5. Reduce heat to low. Add almond butter, coconut milk, honey, fish sauce, vinegar and lime juice. Whisk until blended. Gently simmer for 10 minutes. Remove from heat, but keep warm.
6. Preheat outdoor grill or griddle pan over medium-high heat. Lightly coat with coconut oil.
7. Pierce marinated chicken strips with soaked skewers. Pour some *Satay Sauce* over chicken and brush lightly with marinade brush to coat. Transfer remaining *Satay Sauce* to serving dish.
8. Grill chicken on preheated grill until just cooked through, about 3 minutes per side. Turn over skewers halfway through cooking. Do not overcook.
9. Remove skewers from heat and transfer to serving dish. Serve with *Satay Sauce*.

Saucy Meatballs

Prep Time: 10 minutes

Cook Time: 20 minutes

Servings: 4

INGREDIENTS

32 oz (2 lbs) ground meat (beef, pork, chicken, bison, or any combination)

1/2 cup almond flour

2 eggs

2 teaspoons sesame oil (or coconut or almond oil)

2 garlic cloves

4 large green onions (scallions)

1 teaspoon sesame seeds

1/2 teaspoon ground ginger

Sauce

2/3 cup pure fish sauce (or tamari)

1/4 cup coconut vinegar (or apple cider vinegar)

2 tablespoons raw honey (or agave)

2 garlic cloves

1 teaspoon sesame oil

1 teaspoon ground ginger

DIRECTIONS

1. Preheat oven to 400 degrees F. Line baking sheet with parchment or baking mat.

2. Peel garlic and cut 1 green onion in half. Thinly slice remaining 3 1/2 green onions and set aside.
3. Add garlic, sliced green onions, sesame oil, eggs and ginger to food processor or high-speed blender with. Process until coarsely ground, then transfer to large mixing bowl.
4. Add ground meat and almond flour to bowl and mix well with hands or large wooden spoon. Roll mixture into golf ball sized meatballs with scoop or hands.
5. Place meatballs on prepared sheet pan. Bake for 15 - 20 minutes, until golden brown and cooked through.
6. For *Sauce*, peel and mince garlic. Add to small mixing bowl with fish sauce, vinegar, honey, oil and ginger. Mix well.
7. Remove meatballs from oven. Dip in *Sauce* with mini serving fork or toothpick and transfer to serving dish. Transfer remaining *Sauce* to serving dish.
8. Slice remaining 1/2 green onion. Sprinkle sesame seeds and reserved green onions over dish. Serve warm.

Crunchy Cashew Chicken

Prep Time: 10 minutes

Cook Time: 15 minutes

Servings: 4

INGREDIENTS

16 oz (1 lb) boneless, skinless chicken

1 cup raw cashews

1/4 cup cashew butter

1 cage-free egg

Pinch cayenne pepper (optional)

1/4 teaspoon Chinese 5-spice (optional)

1/4 teaspoon ground ginger

1/4 teaspoon garlic powder

1/2 teaspoon ground black pepper

1 teaspoon Celtic sea salt

Bacon fat or coconut oil (for cooking)

Water

INSTRUCTIONS

1. Heat large skillet or pan over medium-high heat. Add 1 - 2 tablespoons bacon fat or coconut oil to hot pan.
2. Add cashews to food processor or high-speed blender. Process until finely chopped or coarsely ground, about 1 minute. Transfer half of cashews to shallow dish.

3. Process remaining cashew until finely ground into flour, about 2 minutes. Transfer cashew flour to separate shallow dish.
4. Add cashew butter and egg to third shallow dish. Mix well to combine. Add enough water to reach saucy consistency.
5. Cut chicken into 1/2 inch strips. Dredge in cashew flour and toss to coat well. Then dip into egg mixture and toss to coat. Place chicken in chopped cashews and press to coat well.
6. Place chicken in hot oiled pan and cook about 1 - 2 minutes on each side, until golden brown and cooked through. Stir occasionally, careful to maintain coating.
7. Transfer cooked chicken to serving dish and serve hot.

Thai Steamed Mussels

Prep Time: 10 minutes

Cook Time: 10

Servings: 2

INGREDIENTS

2.5 lbs fresh mussels

1/2 can (about 6.5 oz) coconut milk

3 tablespoons dry white wine (or tamari or coconut vinegar)

2 teaspoons Thai red curry paste

1/2 tablespoon pure fish sauce

1/2 tablespoon raw honey (or agave)

2 garlic cloves

1 bunch fresh cilantro

2 limes

INSTRUCTIONS

1. Have fishmonger clean mussels. Or scrub mussels and remove the beards with pliers yourself, if necessary.
2. Juice limes into large pot with lid. Peel and mince garlic. Add to pot with coconut milk, wine, curry paste, fish sauce and honey. Heat over high heat and bring to boil. Stir frequently.
3. Simmer for 1 minute, then add mussels. Cover with lid and cook until mussels open, about 5 - 8 minutes. Sir occasionally.
4. Remove from heat. Chop cilantro and toss with mussels.
5. Transfer mussels and liquid to serving dish. Serve hot.

Steak and Eggs

Prep Time: 5 minutes
Cook Time: 20 minutes
Servings: 1

INGREDIENTS

8 oz (1/2 lb) grass-fed bone-in steak (about 1 inch thick)
2 cage-free eggs
Celtic sea salt, to taste
Cracked black pepper, to taste
Coconut oil or bacon fat (for cooking)

INSTRUCTIONS

1. Heat cast iron pan or skillet over medium heat.
2. Sprinkle steak with salt and cracked black pepper on both sides. Place in hot pan and sear about 5 - 7 minutes per side for medium doneness. Flip steak halfway through cooking.
3. Remove steak from hot pan and allow to rest on cutting board or plate for a few minutes.
4. Heat medium pan over medium-high heat. Add 1 heaping tablespoon bacon fat or coconut oil to hot pan.
5. Gently add eggs to hot oiled pan and cover with well fitting lid. Decrease heat to medium-low and let eggs cook about 3 minutes for over-medium doneness.

6. Carefully release eggs from pan with spatula and transfer to serving dish. Top with cracked black pepper, to taste. Transfer rested steak to serving dish and serve hot.

Primal Chicken and Waffles

Prep Time: 20 minutes

Cook Time: 15 minutes

Servings: 2

INGREDIENTS

Waffles

1 cup almond flour

1/4 coconut flour

3 cage-free eggs (separated)

1/4 cup coconut oil (or coconut or cacao butter, melted)

1/4 cup raw honey (or agave, date butter or stevia)

2 teaspoons aluminum-free baking soda

1 teaspoon vanilla

Pinch Celtic sea salt

Coconut oil (for cooking)

Raw honey, agave, fruit syrup (for garnish, optional)

Chicken Strips

8 oz (1/2 lb) boneless, skinless chicken (white or dark meat)

1 cage-free egg

1/2 cup coarse almond meal (or almond flour)

1 teaspoon flax meal

1/2 teaspoon paprika

1/2 teaspoon ground black pepper

1/2 teaspoon Celtic sea salt

1/4 teaspoon cayenne pepper (optional)

INSTRUCTIONS

1. Preheat waffle iron. Use wadded paper towel to carefully coat cooking surface with coconut oil. Heat medium pan over medium-high heat. Lightly coat pan with coconut oil.
2. For *Waffles*, in medium mixing bowl, beat egg whites to medium-stiff peaks with hand mixer, about 5 minutes.
3. In small mixing bowl, combine flours, salt and baking soda. In large mixing bowl, beat together egg yolks, oil or butter, sweetener and vanilla with hand mixer or whisk.
4. Beat flour mixture into egg yolk mixture. Gently fold egg whites into egg yolk batter.
5. Pour portion of batter onto hot waffle iron. Do not overfill. Cook 4 - 5 minutes, until golden brown and crisp. Repeat with remaining batter. Set aside cooked *Waffles*.
6. For *Chicken Strips*, cut chicken into equal portions. Add almond meal, flax meal, salt spices and to shallow dish and blend.
7. Add egg to separate shallow dish and beat. Dip and coat chicken in beaten egg, then dredge and coat well in almond meal mixture.
8. Carefully place coated chicken in hot oiled pan. Cook until golden brown and cooked through, about 3 - 4 minutes per side, depending on thickness. Turn with tongs halfway through cooking.
9. Remove *Chicken Strips* from pan and place on paper towel to drain.

10. Transfer cooked *Waffles* to serving dish. Top with *Chicken Strips*. Drizzle with raw honey, agave, or your favorite fruit syrup (optional).
11. Serve immediately.

Southern Style Egg Salad

Prep Time: 5 minutes

Cook Time: 15 minutes

Servings: 4

INGREDIENTS

8 cage-free eggs

1 avocado

1 celery stalk

1/4 sweet onion

1/4 cup sweet pickle relish (or dill pickle relish + 1 tablespoon raw honey, agave or date butter)

1/4 cup organic mustard

2 teaspoons paprika

1/2 teaspoon ground black pepper

1/4 teaspoon Celtic sea salt

INSTRUCTIONS

1. Bring medium pot of lightly salted water to a boil. Leave enough room in pot for eggs.
2. Gently add eggs to hot water with tongs and cook about 10 minutes.
3. Drain eggs into colander in sink. Fill pot with cold water and add eggs back to pot. Let cold water run slowly over eggs in pot to cool.

4. Slice and pit avocado. Scoop flesh into medium mixing bowl. Thinly slice celery. Peel and finely dice onion. Add to mixing bowl with relish, mustard, salt and spices. Mix with large spoon to combine.
5. Crack cooled eggs and peel off shells. Add boiled eggs to medium mixing bowl.
6. Use a fork or knife to chop eggs. Use large spoon to mix and mash ingredients together until smooth mixture with soft chunks forms. Stir to combine.
7. Transfer to serving dish and serve immediately. Or refrigerate about 20 minutes and serve chilled.

Meaty Texas Chili

Prep Time: 5 minutes

Cook Time: 40 minutes

Servings: 4

INGREDIENTS

16 oz (1 lb) lean grass-fed ground beef (or elk, bison, turkey or chicken)

15 oz (1 can) organic tomato sauce

29 oz (2 cans) organic diced tomatoes

1 cup water

1 cup cashews

1 small onion

1 bell pepper

2 cloves garlic

2 tablespoons chili powder

1 1/2 tablespoons smoked paprika (or paprika)

1 tablespoon ground cumin

1 teaspoon Mexican oregano (or dried oregano)

1 teaspoon ground black pepper

1/2 teaspoon cayenne pepper

1 teaspoon Celtic sea salt

1 tablespoon coconut oil

INSTRUCTIONS

1. Heat medium pot over medium-high heat. Add 1 tablespoon coconut oil to hot pan.

2. Peel onion and garlic. Remove stems, seeds and veins from bell pepper. Roughly chop and add to food processor or high-speed blender. Pulse until finely minced.
3. Add minced veggies to hot skillet and sauté for about 1 minute. Add ground beef and spices. Brown beef for about 5 minutes. Stir with whisk to break up meat well, or wooden spoon to keep beef chunkier.
4. Add whole cans of diced tomatoes and tomato sauce, and water. Stir to combine.
5. Bring to a simmer, then reduce heat to medium and cover pot loosely with lid to prevent splatter. Simmer about 30 minutes. Stir occasionally.
6. Remove from heat and transfer to serving dish. Use large serving spoon or ladle to serve hot.

Almond Crust Chicken Pie

Prep Time: 25 minutes*

Cook Time: 45 minutes

Servings: 4

INGREDIENTS

Filling

16oz (1lb) boneless skin-on chicken (or pheasant, game hen, etc.)

2 cups chicken broth

2 large carrots

1 large celery stalk

1 green bell pepper

1 small onion

2 garlic cloves

1/2 lemon

1 cage-free egg

2 tablespoons tapioca flour

2 tablespoons coconut flour

2 teaspoons dried thyme (or 4 teaspoons fresh thyme)

1/2 teaspoon black pepper

Celtic sea salt (to taste)

Bacon fat or coconut oil (for cooking)

Crust

1 1/2 cup almond flour

1/2 cup coconut flour

3/4 cup cold coconut oil (or room temperature cacao butter)

3 cage-free eggs

2 teaspoons dried thyme

1 teaspoon Celtic sea salt

Water

INSTRUCTIONS

1. *For *Crust*, add almond and coconut flour, thyme and salt to medium mixing bowl. Cut oil or butter into flour with fork until crumbly. Mix in eggs until dough starts to combine together. Mix in enough water to bring together tender dough.
2. *Divide dough in half and roll into round disks. Place one dough round over pie pan or plate and gentle press in. Cover and place in freezer 1 hour. Cover and refrigerate remaining dough.
3. Preheat oven to 350 degrees F. Heat large pot over medium heat.
4. For *Filling*, add 2 tablespoons bacon fat or coconut oil to hot pot. Add chicken pieces skin-side down. Cook chicken until browned and fat renders out, about 5 minutes. Turn chicken over and continue cooking another 5 minutes. Remove chicken from pot and set aside.
5. Add coconut and tapioca flour to pot and whisk until smooth paste forms. Gradually whisk in chicken broth. Simmer about 5 minutes, whisking occasionally.

Nuts & Turkey Burgers

Prep time: 10 minutes

Cook time: 6-12 minutes

Servings: 4

INGREDIENTS

16 oz ground turkey

1 cup walnuts

2 cloves garlic

1 onion

¼ tsp chipotle chili pepper powder

¼ tbsp smoked paprika

¼ tsp ground black pepper

INSTRUCTIONS

1. Chop walnuts into smaller pieces, about ⅛" cubes. Mince garlic and chop onion into small pieces, about ¼" pieces.
2. Combine the above with ground turkey and add chipotle chili pepper powder, smoked paprika and ground black pepper. Knead it all together and separate into four patties.
3. Cook on the grill on high heat, flipping occasionally, until desired done-ness.

Baked Tilapia Filets

Prep time: 10 minutes

Cook time: 15 minutes

Serves: 4

INGREDIENTS

4 filets of tilapia

¼ tsp chipotle chili pepper powder

1 lemon

1 cup coconut milk

1 clove garlic

1 tsp lemon juice

2 tbsp dill

¼ tsp black ground pepper

INSTRUCTIONS

1. Preheat oven to 350 degrees. Chop the garlic and the dill and cut the lemon into slices.
2. Season tilapia with chipotle chili pepper powder and black ground pepper. Bake for 15 minutes or until tilapia flakes with a fork.
3. Combine coconut milk, garlic, lemon juice and dill in a bowl.

4. Remove fish from oven and pour sauce over the top, placing a lemon wedge over each. Serve immediately or chill 20 minutes and then serve.

Super Simple Protein Matzo Ball Soup

Prep Time: 5 minutes*
Cook Time: 10 minutes
Servings: 6

INGREDIENTS

6 cups chicken stock (or vegetable stock)
2 cups almond flour
4 cage-free egg yolks
1/4 teaspoon ground white pepper (or ground black pepper)
2 teaspoons Celtic sea salt

INSTRUCTIONS

1. In a medium bowl, beat eggs, 1 teaspoon salt and pepper until light and frothy, about 2 minutes. Sift almond flour into bowl and mix until dough comes together.
2. *Cover dough with parchment, if preferred, and refrigerate 2 - 4 hours.
3. Add 1 teaspoon salt to large pot of water and bring to boil. Add chicken stock to medium pot and heat over medium heat.
4. Remove dough from refrigerator and roll into balls. Carefully place dough balls in boiling water. Reduce heat to low, cover and simmer 20 minutes, until cooked through.
5. Transfer matzo balls to serving dish with slotted spoon. Ladle heated chicken stock over matzo balls and serve hot.

Highland Beef Haggis

Prep Time: 10 minutes

Cook Time: 3 hours

Servings: 4

INGREDIENTS

8 oz (1/2 lb) ground beef (or bison, elk, etc.)

8 oz (1/2 lb) lamb shoulder

4 oz (1/4 lb) calves liver

2 onions (yellow or white)

1/2 head cauliflower (about 1 cup riced)

1 cup beef stock

2 garlic cloves

1/2 teaspoon ground nutmeg

1/4 teaspoon ground coriander

1/2 teaspoon Celtic sea salt

1/2 ground white pepper (or ground black pepper)

1/4 cup ghee (or coconut oil or cacao butter)

Water

INSTRUCTIONS

1. Preheat oven to 300 degrees F. Generously coat baking dish with ghee, oil or butter.
2. Add liver to small pan with enough water to cover over high heat. Bring to simmer and cook about 5 minutes. Drain and set aside to cool.

3. Roughly chop cauliflower. Peel and roughly chop onions and garlic. Add to food processor with lamb shoulder and par-cooked liver. Process until coarsely ground, about 2 minutes.
4. Add ground beef, stock, salt, and spices and pulse to combine. Transfer to prepared baking dish and cover tightly with aluminum foil.
5. Place covered dish in roasting pan. Add water to roasting pan 3/4 of the way up side of baking dish.
6. Bake for 3 hours. Remove from oven and carefully remove foil. Let rest about 10 minutes.
7. Remove baking dish from roasting pan. To plate, place serving dish over baking dish and carefully invert. Slice haggis into wedges and serve hot with mashed parsnips or yams.

Bacon Wrapped Filet Mignon

Prep Time: 5 minutes
Cook Time: 20 minutes
Servings: 2

INGREDIENTS

2 (6 oz each) filet mignon steaks
2 thick slices nitrate-free bacon
Ground black pepper, to taste
Celtic sea salt, to taste
1 tablespoon coconut oil (optional)
Toothpicks

INSTRUCTIONS

1. Preheat oven to 350 degrees F. Heat medium oven-safe pan or skillet over medium heat.
2. Add bacon to hot pan. Cook and render out fat for about 5 minutes, until about halfway cooked. Remove bacon from pan and set aside, reserving bacon fat in pan. Add coconut oil to pan, if desired.
3. Wrap par-cooked bacon around steaks and secure with toothpick. Sprinkle steaks with salt and pepper to taste.
4. Add wrapped seasoned steaks to hot oiled pan and sear 2 minutes per side. Carefully flip half way through cooking.
5. Remove pan from stove and place in preheated oven. Cook about 8 - 10 minutes, until bacon is cooked through and steak is medium-rare.

6. Remove steaks from oven and transfer to cutting board. Set aside and let rest at least 2 minutes.
7. Transfer to serving dish and serve hot.

Herb Crusted Pork Chops with Cinnamon Apples

Prep Time: 10 minutes
Cook Time: 30 minutes
Servings: 4

INGREDIENTS

Pork Chops

4 pork chops (bone-in or boneless)

1/2 cup almond flour

2 tablespoons coconut oil (or cacao butter or ghee)

1 sprig fresh rosemary

1 teaspoon dried thyme

Ground black pepper, to taste

Celtic sea salt, to taste

Coconut oil (for cooking)

Cinnamon Apples

4 tart apples

1/4 cup raw honey (or agave or date butter)

1 tablespoon ground cinnamon

2 tablespoons coconut oil (or cacao butter or ghee)

INSTRUCTIONS

1. Preheat oven to 350 degrees F. Heat large pan over medium heat. Add 2 tablespoons oil, butter or ghee to hot pan.
2. Lightly coat wire rack or slotted broiler pan with coconut oil. Place over sheet pan layered with aluminum foil to catch drippings.
3. For *Pork Chops*, pat pork chops dry and sprinkle with salt and pepper. Place on wire rack or broiler pan.
4. Remove rosemary needles from stem and chop. Add to small mixing bowl with almond flour, coconut oil, thyme, salt and pepper. Mix to form paste.
5. Press seasoned paste into top of each pork chop with fingers to form a 1/8 inch thick crust.
6. Place pork chops in oven and bake about 20 - 25 minutes.
7. For *Cinnamon Apples*, peel and core apple. Cut apples into thick slices and add to large mixing bowl with sweetener and cinnamon. Mix to combine.
8. Add seasoned apples to hot oiled pan. Sauté about 5 minutes, until aromatic and lightly browned. Reduce heat to medium-low and add 1/2 cup water.
9. Cover pan with lid or aluminum foil and simmer about 20 minutes, or until apples are tender. Stir occasionally.
10. Set oven to BROIL and move pork chops about 6 inches away from the heating element. Broil for about 5 minutes, until topping is browned. Rotate halfway through broiling, if necessary. Do not burn topping.
11. Transfer *Cinnamon Apples* to serving dish. Remove pork chops from oven and place over *Cinnamon Apples*.
12. Serve immediately.

Sausage Stuffed Tomatoes

Prep Time: 10 minutes

Cook Time: 40 minutes

Servings: 4

INGREDIENTS

8 small-medium tomatoes (red, yellow, green, or any combination)

16 oz (1 lb) Italian sausage (sweet or spicy)

1 celery stalk

1/2 onion (white or yellow)

1/2 cup red radishes (about 6)

1/2 cup walnuts (or pecans, almonds, etc.)

1/3 cup nutritional yeast (optional)

6 large basil leaves basil

1 tablespoon fresh thyme leaves

Celtic sea salt, to taste

Ground black pepper, to taste

2 tablespoons bacon fat (or coconut oil)

INSTRUCTIONS

1. Preheat oven to 350 degrees F.
2. Cut tops off tomatoes, then remove stems from tops and seeds and juices from bottoms of tomatoes. Leave bottoms of tomatoes hollow but do not pierce. Place in baking dish just large enough to fit tomatoes snuggly. Set aside.

3. Peel onion and garlic. Mince or coarsely grate garlic, onion and radish. Finely dice celery and tops of tomatoes. Finely chop basil and thyme leaves. Coarsely chop pecans. Add to medium mixing bowl with sausage, salt and pepper to taste, and nutritional yeast (optional). Mix well.
4. Use large spoon to stuff tomatoes with mixture. Drizzle bacon fat or coconut oil over tomatoes. Cover tomatoes with aluminum foil.
5. Bake 25 minutes. Carefully remove foil and continue baking uncovered 10 - 15 minutes, until stuffing is golden brown.
6. Carefully remove from oven and serve hot.

Stuffed Cabbage in Tomato Sauce

Prep Time: 15 minutes

Cook Time: 60 minutes

Servings: 6

INGREDIENTS

1 large cabbage head

Filling

2 1/2 lbs ground beef

4 cage-free eggs

1/2 onion (yellow or white)

1/3 cup almond flour

1/2 cup cauliflower (riced or minced)

1/2 teaspoon dried thyme

1/2 teaspoon ground black pepper (or ground white pepper)

1 1/2 teaspoons Celtic sea salt

Tomato Sauce

2 cans (15 oz) organic tomato sauce

1/2 cup golden raisins

1/2 onion (yellow or white)

2 tablespoons raw honey (or agave or date butter)

2 tablespoons apple cider vinegar

1 1/2 teaspoons Celtic sea salt

1 teaspoon ground black pepper (or ground white pepper)

2 tablespoons bacon fat (or coconut oil or ghee)

INSTRUCTIONS

1. Preheat oven to 350 degrees F. Bring large pot of salted water to boil.
2. Carefully place cabbage head in boiling water for about 5 minutes. Use tongs to peel each layer of leaves from head as soon as they become tender. Set leaves aside on sheet pan to cool.
3. For *Tomato Sauce*, peel and mince onions. Add 1/2 of onions to medium mixing bowl. Add tomato sauce, honey, vinegar, raisins, salt and spices and mix to combine.
4. For *Filling*, add remaining onions to large mixing bowl. Mince or rice cauliflower and add to bowl with eggs, almond flour, salt, spices, and 1 cup *Tomato Sauce*. Mix well with hands or large wooden spoon.
5. Cut hard rib from bottom of each cooled cabbage leaf. Place 1/3 - 1/2 cup *Filling* near the bottom edge of cabbage leaf and roll into a neat package, tucking in sides as you roll. Repeat with remaining filling and cabbage.
6. Spread 1 cup *Tomato sauce* along bottom of deep, lidded baking dish. Place 1/2 the cabbage rolls in baking dish. Add 1/2 remaining sauce, the remaining cabbage rolls. Top with remaining sauce.
7. Tightly cover dish with lid and bake for 1 hour, until meat is cooked through and veggies are tender.
8. Transfer to serving dish and serve hot.

Beef Burgundy

Prep Time: 30 minutes
Cook Time: 7 hours
Servings: 6

INGREDIENTS

3 lbs boneless stew beef
2 cups beef stock (or broth)
1 bottle (750 ml) organic dry red wine
1/2 cup organic sparkling apple cider (or cognac)
8 oz (1/2 lb) nitrate-free bacon
1 pint fresh mushrooms (about 2 cups)
4 large carrots
2 yellow onions
2 cups whole pearl onions (peeled)
2 garlic cloves
1 tablespoon organic tomato paste
3 tablespoons tapioca flour (arrowroot powder)
1/2 teaspoon dried thyme
1 teaspoon ground black pepper
2 teaspoons Celtic sea salt
2 tablespoons coconut oil (for cooking)

INSTRUCTIONS

1. Heat large skillet over medium-high heat. Add coconut oil to hot pan.

2. Cut beef into chunks than add to large mixing bowl. Season beef with salt and pepper, then add 2 tablespoons tapioca or arrowroot. Toss to coat.
3. Add seasoned beef to hot oiled pan in batches to brown, about 5 minutes per batch. Set aside in slow cooker.
4. Chop bacon and add to hot pan. Sauté until just crisp and fat renders out, about 5 - 8 minutes. Set aside in slow cooker.
5. Peel and chop yellow onions. Peel and mince garlic. Add to hot bacon grease and sauté about 5 minutes. Set aside in slow cooker.
6. Cut mushrooms in half. Add to hot pan with tomato paste, remaining tapioca or arrow root, thyme and apple cider. Stir to combine. Then add beef stock to deglaze pan. Bring to simmer, about 5 minutes.
7. Pour mushroom mixture into slow cooker. Add red wine and peeled pearl onions. Chop carrots and add to slow cooker. Stir to combine.
8. Cover slow cooker with lid. Turn on to low and cook 6 - 8 hours, until meat and veggies are tender.
9. Turn off slow cooker and carefully remove lid.
10. Transfer to serving dish and serve hot.

Delicious Lobster Bisque

Prep Time: 25 minutes
Cook Time: 40 minutes
Servings: 4

INGREDIENTS

16 oz (1 lb) lobster meat (claws and tail from 2 - 3 lobsters)
4 cups vegetable broth
1 can (13.5 oz) full-fat coconut milk (or lite coconut milk)
1 can (6 oz) organic tomato paste
2 tablespoons coconut aminos (apple cider vinegar or liquid aminos)
2 leeks
2 carrots
2 celery stalks
4 large garlic cloves
2 bay leaves
1/2 teaspoon dried basil
1/2 teaspoon dried thyme
1 teaspoon dried oregano
1 teaspoon fresh cracked black pepper (or ground black pepper)
Celtic sea salt, to taste
1 small bunch freash parsley (for garnish)
2 tablespoons ghee (or bacon fat, cacao butter, or coconut oil)

INSTRUCTIONS

1. Chop leeks, carrots and celery. Peel garlic and chop. Add to medium pot with vegetable broth, oregano, basil, thyme, pepper and salt to taste. Add tomato paste and stir to combine. Simmer about 25 minutes.
2. Bring large pot salted water to boil. Boil each lobster about 2 minutes. Let cool, then crack shells and remove meat from claws and tail. Roughly chop and set aside.
3. Pour veggies and broth into food processor or high-speed blender. Process until puréed, about 2 minutes.
4. Add puréed mixture back to pot and heat over medium heat. Bring to simmer and add chopped lobster meat. Stir to combine. Simmer until lobster is cooked through and tender, about 10 minutes.
5. Transfer to serving dish and serve hot.

Stewed Chicken and Dumplings

Prep Time: 10 minutes

Cook Time: 1 hour 20 minutes

Servings: 4

INGREDIENTS

2 lb whole chicken (innards removed)

6 - 10 cups water

3 carrots

3 celery stalks

1 small white onion (or yellow onion)

4 bay leaves

1 1/2 tablespoons dried thyme (or 4 sprigs fresh thyme)

1/2 teaspoon dried oregano

1 teaspoon paprika

2 teaspoon ground black pepper

1 tablespoon Celtic sea salt

Dumplings

3 cups almond flour

1/2 cup arrowroot powder

2 cage-free egg

1/2 cup coconut oil, chilled (or coconut or cacao butter, room temperature)

1/2 teaspoon baking soda

1/4 teaspoon ground bay leaf

1 teaspoon dried thyme

1/2 teaspoon ground white pepper (or ground black pepper)

1 teaspoon Celtic sea salt

Nut milk (or chicken broth or stock)

INSTRUCTIONS

1. Heat large pot over medium-high heat. Place chicken breast-down in hot pot. Sear chicken and turn to brown and render out fat for about 15 minutes.
2. Chop carrots and celery. Peel onion and mince. Add to chicken with salt and spices. Sauté about 2 minutes.
3. Add enough water to pot to cover chicken. Increase heat to high and bring to a boil. Reduce heat to medium and simmer about 30 minutes. Place lid loosely over pot to prevent splatter, if necessary.
4. For *Dumplings*, sift almond flour and arrowroot into medium mixing bowl. Cut in solid oil or butter with fork until crumbly mixture forms. Add egg, salt and spices, baking soda, and enough nut milk or chicken broth from pot to bring together soft, slightly sticky dough.
5. Carefully remove chicken from pot with long utensil and set aside. Use utensils to remove skin from chicken. Carve chicken into desired pieces and place back in back.
6. Use spoon or scoop to gently drop dough into pot. Cover with well fitting lid and let simmer about 15 - 20 minutes, until *Dumplings* and chicken are cooked through. Gently stir soup to periodically prevent *Dumplings* from sticking. Turn over any *Dumplings* that are not submerged.
7. Remove from heat and transfer to serving dish. Serve hot.

Macadamia Crusted Ahi Tuna

Prep Time: 5 minutes

Cook Time: 1 minute

Servings: 1

INGREDIENTS

8 oz ahi tuna fillet

1/4 teaspoon coconut oil

1/4 teaspoon dried thyme

1/4 teaspoon dried tarragon (optional)

1/4 cup whole macadamia nuts (shelled)

1 small garlic clove teaspoon

1 small shallot teaspoon

1/2 teaspoon ground white pepper (or black pepper)

1/2 teaspoon sea salt

2 tablespoons coconut oil

INSTRUCTIONS

1. Heat medium pan over medium-high heat. Add 2 tablespoons coconut oil to pan.
2. Chop macadamia nuts well. Peel and finely mince garlic and shallot. Set aside.
3. Rub top and bottom of fillet with 1/4 teaspoon coconut oil, salt, pepper, thyme and tarragon (optional).
4. Press 1/2 chopped macadamia nuts into each side of fillet.

5. Add garlic and shallots to hot oiled pan and sauté for just a second. Do not burn.
6. Carefully place fish in pan and sear 15 - 30 seconds on each side, for rare to medium rare. Carefully flip half way through cooking.
7. Transfer fillet to serving dish and serve hot with mixed greens or favorite veggies.

Lobster Newburg

Prep Time: 15 minutes

Cook Time: 25 minutes

Servings: 6

INGREDIENTS

2 (1 lb) live lobsters

2 egg yolks

1/2 cup coconut cream (or kefir + 2 tablespoons sweetener*)

1/4 cup ghee (or cacao butter)

2 tablespoons dry sherry (or 1 tablespoon apple cider vinegar + 1 teaspoon sweetener*)

1/2 teaspoon sea salt

1/4 teaspoon cayenne pepper

1 /4 teaspoon ground nutmeg

Biscuits

1 1/4 cups almond flour

1 egg

2 tablespoons coconut oil

3/4 teaspoon baking soda

1/8 teaspoon ground white pepper

1/4 teaspoon sea salt

INSTRUCTIONS

1. Preheat oven to 350 degrees F. Line sheet pan with parchment paper. Place 4 ceramic ramekins on parchment, and lightly coat bottom with coconut oil.
2. Bring large pot of salted water to boil. Use tongs to carefully place each lobster in boiling water for just 1 minute. Remove from pot. Crack lobster claws and tails and remove meat. Roughly chop, and set aside.
3. For *Biscuits*, separate egg white into medium bowl, and add yolk to small bowl with coconut oil.
4. Beat egg whites to soft peaks with hand mixer or whisk. Mix yolk and oil, almond flour, baking soda, salt and pepper into egg white to form soft, solid dough.
5. Roll dough into eight balls, then flatten into 1/2-inch thick round biscuits with hands. They should fit ramekins snuggly. Place 1 biscuit at bottom of each ramekin. Set remaining biscuits aside on parchment sheet next to ramekins.
6. In small bowl, whisk together egg yolks and coconut cream until well blended.
7. Melt ghee in medium pan over low heat. Stir in egg mixture and sherry. Stir and cook until mixture thickens slightly, about 5 minutes.
8. Add salt, cayenne and nutmeg. Add par cooked lobster meat and cook about 1 minute then remove from heat.
9. Scoop portion of lobster mixture into each ramekin, over biscuit. Top with remaining biscuit.
10. Place sheet pan in oven and bake 15 minutes, until biscuit is golden and firm on top.

11. Remove from oven and let cool slightly.
12. Serve warm.

raw honey or agave nectar

Island Lamb Patty

Prep Time: 25 minutes

Cook Time: 30 minutes

Servings: 4

INSTRUCTIONS

Crust

2 cups almond flour

2 cage-free eggs

1/4 cup ghee (or coconut butter, cacao butter, or chilled coconut oil)

1 teaspoon turmeric (optional)

1/4 teaspoon paprika (optional)

1/4 teaspoon baking soda

1/2 teaspoon Celtic sea salt

Filling

12 oz (3/4 lb) ground lamb

1/2 small onion (yellow, white or red)

1 tablespoon tamari (or coconut aminos)

1 tablespoon raw honey (or agave or date butter)

1 tablespoon curry powder

1 teaspoon allspice

1 teaspoon chili powder

1 teaspoon red pepper flake

1/2 teaspoon garlic powder

1/2 teaspoon onion powder

1/2 teaspoon Celtic sea salt

INSTRUCTIONS
1. For *Crust*, sift almond flour into medium mixing bowl. Add baking soda, salt and spices (optional).
2. Whisk eggs in small mixing bowl, then add to flour and combine. Slowly cut in coconut oil with fork until malleable dough comes together.
3. Roll dough in plastic wrap or wrap tightly in parchment and refrigerate for 15 minutes.
4. Preheat oven to 400 degrees F. Line sheet pan with parchment or baking mat. Cover cutting board with parchment. Heat medium pan over medium heat.
5. For *Filling*, peel and mince or finely grate onion. Add onion and ground lamb to hot pan with salt and spices. Sauté until lamb is browned and onions are soft, about 8 minutes. Remove from heat and set aside.
6. Remove dough from refrigerator and divide into 4 portions. Roll dough into balls and use hands to flatten on prepared cutting board. Roll into circles about 1/8 inch thick with rolling pin.
7. Scoop equal portions of *Filling* into center of one half of dough circle. Fold bare half of dough over filled half. Press edges together, letting any trapped air escape. Crimp edges of dough together with fork. Repeat with remaining dough.
8. Arrange patties on lined sheet pan and bake 15 - 20 minutes, until dough is golden and cooked through.

9. Remove from oven and transfer *Patties* to wire rack to cool completely. Once cooled, place in airtight container and store in freezer. Place small parchment sheets in between patties, if desired.
10. To serve, place patties in toaster, toaster oven or preheated oven and cook until heated through.

Jamaican Curried Goat

Prep Time: 30 minutes*

Cook Time: 5 hours

Servings: 6

INGREDIENTS

3 lb goat or lamb (boneless or bone-in)

2 cans (14 oz) full-fat coconut milk

1 can (15 oz) organic tomato sauce (or crushed tomatoes)

5 large parsnips

2 onions (yellow or white)

1 chili pepper (habañero, scotch bonnet, etc.)

2 inch piece fresh ginger

4 garlic cloves

6 tablespoons Jamaican curry powder (or 6 tablespoons curry powder + 1 tablespoon allspice)

1 tablespoon dried thyme

1 tablespoon Celtic sea salt

1/4 cup coconut oil (for cooking)

1 - 2 cups water

INSTRUCTIONS

1. *Season goat with salt and set aside in baking dish until room temperature, about up to 30 minutes.
2. Heat large skillet over medium-high heat. Add coconut oil to hot pan.

3. Peel and chop onions. Peel and mince garlic and ginger. Remove stem and seeds from chili pepper, then finely chop. Cut goat into chunks.
4. Add 2 tablespoon curry powder to hot oil. Add goat to hot seasoned oil in batches to brown, about 5 minutes per batch. Set aside in slow cooker.
5. Add onions and chili pepper to hot pan. Sauté until just golden and fragrant, about 5 - 8 minutes. Add garlic and ginger. Sauté about 1 minute.
6. Add onion mixture and remaining curry powder to slow cooker. Add tomato sauce, coconut milk and water. Stir to combine.
7. Cover slow cooker with lid. Turn on to high and cook about 4 hours, until just tender but not done.
8. Roughly chop parsnips and add to slow cooker. Cover with liquid. Continue cooking about 1 hour, until meat and veggies are tender.
9. Turn off slow cooker and carefully remove lid. Skim off any fat from surface and remove any bones.
10. Transfer to serving dish and serve hot.

Holiday Baked Ham

Prep Time: 10 minutes

Cook Time: 5 hours

Servings: 12

INGREDIENTS

1 (12 lb) bone-in ham

1 (20 oz) can organic pineapple rings (in juice)

1/2 cup date butter (or raw honey or agave)

1/2 cup whole cloves

1/2 cup water

1 lemon

1 lime

1 orange

About 12 pitted cherries (optional)

Toothpicks (optional)

INSTRUCTIONS

1. Preheat oven to 325 degrees F.
2. Drain pineapple juice into small mixing bowl. Juice lemon, lime and orange into bowl. Add sweetener and water. Mix well.
3. Place ham in roasting pan and score rind in crosshatch (diamond) pattern with knife.
4. Press cloves into rind. Place cherries on rind and secure with toothpick. Hang pineapple rings on cherries.

5. Pour pineapple juice mixture over ham and bake uncovered 4 - 5 hours, until internal temperature reaches 160 degrees F. Baste with juices about every 30 minutes.
6. Remove ham from oven. Remove toothpicks and carve. Serve hot.

Chickplant Filets

Prep time: 10 minutes

Cook time: 50 minutes

Serves: 4

INGREDIENTS

4 grass-fed chicken breasts

1 eggplant

4 pinches fresh basil

¼ tsp chipotle chili pepper powder

¼ tsp curry

1 large carrot

1 red onion

1 cup coconut milk

8 wooden toothpicks

1 tbsp coconut oil

INSTRUCTIONS

1. Cut eggplant into 8 rectangles 3" long by 1" wide and 1" tall. Cut the carrot into matchsticks and dice the onion into small pieces. Cut the chicken in half lengthwise into thin filets. Soak the toothpicks in water. Preheat oven to 350.
2. Combine coconut oil, carrot, onion, 1 tsp curry, basil and chipotle chili pepper powder in a pan over medium heat. Stir together until it forms a sauce. Add eggplant and saute 7-10 minutes or until eggplant is tender.

3. Place 1 slice of eggplant on each of the chicken filets. Drizzle the contents of the pan over each of the filets; roll each fillet up around the eggplant and secure with a toothpick.
4. Place the 8 filets in the oven and bake for 35 minutes.
5. Remove from oven and pour serve 2 filets to each plate. Pour ¼ cup coconut milk and sprinkle curry over each plate's filets. Chill 20 minutes and then serve.

Salmon with Berry Chutney

Prep time: 10 minutes
Cook time: 15 minutes
Serves: 4

INGREDIENTS
4 salmon filets
16 stalks of asparagus
1 cup blueberries
1 onion
1 clove garlic
1 tbsp ginger root
¼ cup apple cider vinegar
½ tsp cinnamon

INSTRUCTIONS

1. Preheat your broiler. Finely chop the onion, garlic and ginger. Prepare a stove-top pot to steam the asparagus.
2. Combine blueberry, onion, garlic, ginger, apple cider vinegar and cinnamon in a saucepan and bring to a simmer, stirring continuously. Remove from heat once it has thickened into a sauce and set aside to cool.
3. Steam the asparagus for 3-5 minutes and broil the fish for 5-7 minutes. Remove from oven.

4. Lay one piece of fish across each plate and pour the blueberry chutney over top. Lay 4 stalks of asparagus over each piece of fish and serve.

Oven-Fried Chicken

Prep Time: 10 minutes
Cook Time: 60 minutes
Servings: 4

INGREDIENTS

32 oz (2 lb) bone-in, skinless chicken
3/4 cup fine almond flour
3/4 cup coarse almond meal (or almond flour)
2 cage free eggs
1/3 cup nut milk
1/2 teaspoon cayenne pepper
1 teaspoon ground black pepper
1 1/2 teaspoons paprika
1 1/2 tablespoons Celtic sea salt
Coconut oil (in spray bottle)

INSTRUCTIONS

1. Preheat oven to 350 degrees F. Fill spray bottle with warm coconut oil.
2. Line sheet pan with aluminum foil. Place metal cooling or baking rack over lined sheet pan. Generously spray metal rack with coconut oil to coat. Set second sheet pan aside.
3. Add almond meal and/or flour to small mixing bowl with 1 tablespoon salt and spices. Mix to combine with fork or whisk to break up clumps.

4. In shallow dish, beat eggs and nut milk until combined.
5. Use serving spoon or measuring cup to dust second sheet pan with layer of almond flour mixture onto. Sprinkle chicken with 1/2 tablespoon salt.
6. Dip and coat all chicken pieces in egg mixture then lay on second sheet pan, over layer of almond flour mixture. Use spoon or measuring cut to sprinkle almond flour mixture from mixing bowl over dipped chicken. Pat almond flour mixture into chicken on all sides until well coated.
7. Transfer coasted chicken to prepared wire rack. Generously spray coated chicken with coconut oil.
8. Bake 60 - 70 minutes, until coating is crisp and chicken is cooked through. Remove from oven and allow to cool at least 10 minutes. Then place crispy chicken on paper towels to drain, if desired.
9. Transfer to serving dish and serve immediately.

Country Fried Steak

Prep Time: 10 minutes
Cook Time: 15 minutes
Servings: 2

INGREDIENTS

Country Fried Steak

12 oz (3/4 lb) grass-fed beef (cube steak or fillet)
1 cage-free egg
1 teaspoon coconut aminos (or tamari)
1/3 cup arrowroot powder
1/4 cup macadamia nuts
1/4 cup pistachios (or almonds or cashews)
1/4 teaspoon garlic powder
1/4 teaspoon onion powder
1/4 teaspoon paprika
1/4 teaspoon cracked black pepper (or ground black pepper)
1/4 teaspoon Celtic sea salt
Pinch cayenne pepper
Pinch dried oregano
Coconut oil (for cooking)
Bacon fat (for cooking)

White Gravy

2 teaspoons arrowroot powder
5 oz (1/2 can) full-fat coconut milk

1/2 teaspoon Celtic salt

1/2 teaspoon ground white pepper (or ground black pepper)

Bacon fat

INSTRUCTIONS

1. Heat cast iron pan or skillet over medium-high heat. Add 1 tablespoon each bacon fat and coconut oil to hot pan.
2. For *Country Fried Steak*, add nuts to food processor or high-speed blender. Process until finely ground. Add arrowroot, salt and spices. Pulse to incorporated. Transfer mixture to shallow dish. Set aside.
3. In separate shallow dish, beat egg and coconut aminos. Set aside.
4. Tenderize beef fillet with tenderizing mallet, if using. Dip and coat cube steak in egg mixture, then dredge and coat well in nut mixture.
5. Place coated cube steak into hot oiled pan. Cook until golden and crisp, about 2 minutes on each side. Repeat with remaining steak. Remove cooked steak from pan and place on paper towel to drain.
6. For *White Gravy*, add enough bacon fat to hot skillet so there is about 2 - 3 tablespoons in pan. Allow to heat thoroughly.
7. Add arrowroot to pan. Whisk and cook for 1 minute. Whisk in coconut milk. Whisk and cook another minute. Whisk in salt and pepper. Remove from heat.
8. Transfer *Country Fried Steak* to serving dish. Top with *White Gravy* and serve hot.

Southern Liver and Onions

Prep Time: 20 minutes*

Cook Time: 25 minutes

Servings: 4

INGREDIENTS

20 oz (1 1/4 lb) calves liver

2 onions (yellow or white)

4 slices nitrate-free bacon

1 lemon

2 tablespoons arrowroot powder

1/2 teaspoon Celtic sea salt

1/2 teaspoon cracked black pepper (or ground black pepper)

Bacon fat or coconut oil (for cooking)

INSTRUCTIONS

1. *Remove thin outer membrane from liver and slice into 1/4 inch fillets. Add to glass container. Juice lemon into container and toss to coat. Cover well and refrigerate overnight.
2. Heat large cast-iron pan or skillet set over medium heat.
3. Cut bacon lengthwise into long, thin strips. Then cut in thirds crosswise and add to hot pan. Sauté bacon and let crisp, about 5 minutes. Stir occasionally. Decrease heat to medium-low.
4. Peel and thinly slice onions. Add to bacon and sauté until caramelized, about 10 minutes. Stir occasionally. Remove caramelized onions and bacon from pan and set aside.

5. Drain liver fillets in colander in sink. Rinse under running water, then pat dry.
6. In shallow dish, add arrowroot powder, salt and pepper. Mix with fork to combine.
7. Dredge liver slices in arrowroot mixture and shake off excess. Place coated liver fillets on a plate and coat remaining liver fillets.
8. Add 2 tablespoons bacon fat or coconut oil to hot pan. Add single layer of coated liver to hot oiled pan and sear for 1 minute per side. Place liver on paper towel to drain. Repeat with remaining liver.
9. Transfer liver to serving dish. Top with caramelized onions and bacon. Serve immediately .

Made in the USA
Lexington, KY
26 March 2016